PLAYING CHESS
WITH THE
DEVIL

PLAYING CHESS WITH THE DEVIL

One Family's Journey Through ALS

Julie A. Rouse, Ed. D.

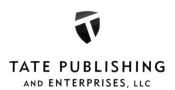

TATE PUBLISHING
AND ENTERPRISES, LLC

Published by Tate Publishing & Enterprises, LLC
127 E. Trade Center Terrace | Mustang, Oklahoma 73064 USA
1.888.361.9473 | www.tatepublishing.com

Tate Publishing is committed to excellence in the publishing industry. The company reflects the philosophy established by the founders, based on Psalm 68:11,
"The Lord gave the word and great was the company of those who published it."

Book design copyright © 2013 by Tate Publishing, LLC. All rights reserved.
Cover design by Joel Uber
Interior design by Mary Jean Archival

Published in the United States of America

ISBN: 978-1-62854-464-0
1. Medical / Diseases
2. Biography & Autobiography / Personal Memoirs
13.07.29

INTRODUCTION

L ife is a series of interruptions. Some are small and require only minor amounts of time, attention, or adjustment. Others are completely life changing and rock us to our core.

December 22, 2003, started out as just another day. As a fourth grade teacher and mother of four young children—then two, six, eight, and twelve—you can imagine the hustle and bustle in the house just three days before Christmas.

My mother called. "The doctors think they know why Dad has been having trouble with his legs. They have diagnosed him with ALS—Lou Gehrig's Disease."

"Oh. What does that mean?"

I had no idea at the time that those words would have such a profound and lasting effect on my life. Of course, the first thing I did after I hung up was begin gathering information about ALS. ALS is categorized into the family of neuromuscular diseases. It is a disease that affects motor neurons in the brain and spinal cord. As these cells slowly die, they stop communicating to muscles to move. As a result, the muscles atrophy or get weaker and smaller. Over time, with no signals from the brain, the muscles in the body continue to weaken and eventually stop working altogether. Doctors are working to try and determine what causes ALS. They are also researching the disease to discover a cure. Currently, there are some promising breakthroughs in research regarding how the disease is contracted and prolonging the quality of life with the use of vitamin supplements and prescription drugs. I truly believed that there would be a cure in time to save my dad's life. He looked healthy except for walking with a cane. He talked, ate, and took care of his hygiene needs on his own. Looking back, I was so naive about everything. I didn't understand what this diagnosis meant, and I didn't understand that research takes the kind of time we didn't have.

ALS can affect people in different ways. Some people begin with their tongue, face, or breathing being affected first. Others experience muscle pain or weakness in one or both arms or legs. Patients who have been diagnosed with ALS typically live for three to five years after being diagnosed with the disease, although my dad lived for nine years. The doctors explained to us that ALS is a disease in which many other diseases first have to be tested for and then ruled out. Through that whole process, the ALS continues to progress.

The next thing I did was search for anything that would give me some insight as to what to expect from this incurable disease. I had the clinical definition from the doctor; I was getting the feeling that this would be a life-changing experience for my whole family, and I was also getting the feeling that traveling the journey of this disease would be similar to walking through thick fog. In retrospect, I wonder if God set it up that way on purpose. I think that sometimes we survive only because we can see just the next step of the journey. If we were to see the entire road, it would be far too overwhelming. A friend suggested *Tuesdays with Morrie* by Mitch Albom, which I voraciously read, through my tears, in one sitting.

Convinced that my father's diagnosis surely wouldn't end that way for us, I continued to search…and found nothing. No blueprint for what would happen next. No instruction manual for me. Panic set in. Sort of like when new parents leave the hospital with that little bundle of joy. Only this time there would be no happy ending.

I wish this disease didn't exist. I wish that books about ALS could have a happy and uplifting tone. Unfortunately, they don't because physically there is no happy and uplifting outcome. The happy and uplifting ending will need to come from a perspective other than that of physical health. If you are reading this book because you (or a family member or friend) have been diagnosed with ALS, I commend you on the journey you are taking. It will change your life more than you ever thought possible. You will find courage and hope in the simplest tasks, visits with friends and family, and in seeing what you are really made of. You are now part of a very close and supportive group of people who will be with you every step of the way if you choose to accept that help and support. I would highly suggest it as this can also be a very lonely and isolated road at times.

I invite you to share the journey my family traveled when my dad, my hero, Jerome "Jerry" Kowalski, was diagnosed. You'll experience our joys, our pain, our anger, and the way my dad taught my sister and me, and our families, about living life and accepting death with grace, humility, and an amazing attitude.

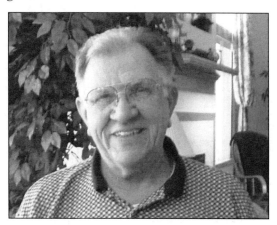

IN THE BEGINNING

My mother and father were married in 1970. She was petite, only 5'1" and about ninety pounds soaking wet. My dad was 6'4" and would easily fill a doorway. He loved and cared for my mom as only a doting husband could. He had his work cut out for him as my mom had a bad heart. In fact, she went into heart failure on their first date, and he had to take her to the emergency room. He said he knew right away that he was destined to take care of her for the rest of her life. That was his story for my sister and me though it had to be difficult. There must have been times where he was less than enthusiastic; although we never knew it. He was a wonderful caretaker to all of us. He wasn't above cooking, cleaning, vacuuming, or doing laundry. He helped care for my sister and me from the time we were born. He had an incredible sense of responsibility, and he loved every minute of it (or at least that's what we believed!).

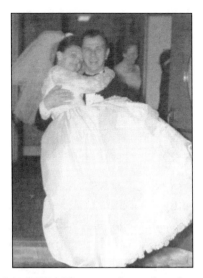

April 11, 1970—The start of something beautiful!

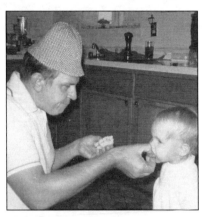

1972—Dad teaching me the fine art of eating a salami sandwich. You have to bite *all the way through*!

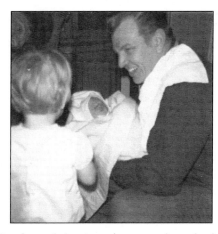

1973—A new baby sister, Ann, completes the family.

Our house was usually happy. From my very early years, I remember going with my dad and sister to drop my mom off to get her hair fixed. We had only one car, so it was a family trip. On the evenings once a week that Mom played bingo, we would spend time together with Dad. We would lie on the living room floor while my dad read stories from the Grimm's Fairy Tales book or other book of our choice. We would play the "Who Can Be the Quietest" game… eventually shortened to "Who Bee's the Quietest," and when my dad would get bored, he'd tickle my sister or me just so one of us would lose, and we could end the game! We played for a slice of pepperoni or peanut M&M's, and we all shared the "winnings," no matter who won.

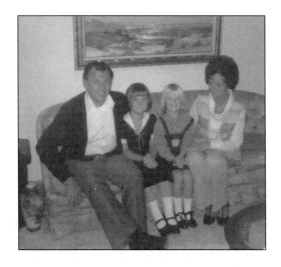

Our house was always full of family and laughter. Mom and Dad were fantastic hosts and loved to entertain. Most holidays found them in the kitchen, cooking up delicious food for extended family and friends. Friends and relatives knew the minute they walked in the house they would have to give their drink order. In fact, it has become well-known through the years that guests should just take something to drink on the first request, even water, because they would be harassed until they finally accepted something! Even my children knew, when they brought their friends to Grandpa and Grandpa's house, to whisper, "Just take a drink. They won't stop asking until you do!"

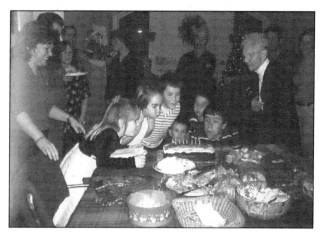

Christmas Eve 2006—Family, food, and happy birthday, Jesus!

Every Christmas and Easter, cousins from far and near would gather at our house to make homemade kielbasa. They would cut the meat by hand, season it with a recipe handed down through the generations, and sit around and share family stories over a beverage or two (well, maybe a few more than that) while the meat marinated. Dad and the senior sausage makers, in the spirit of teasing, would give the new apprentices an initiation, make them sign confidentiality agreements promising to keep the family recipe for seasoning a secret and overall keep them laughing and rolling their eyes through the entire two-day ordeal.

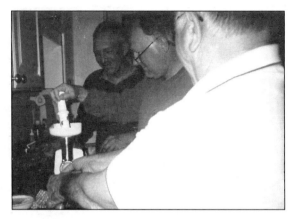

Sausage-making with some of the original
experts: John, Joe, and Dad!

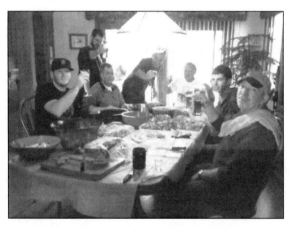

Christmas 2012—A toast to you, Jerry! We'll carry on
the family tradition with our new apprentices!

One year, Mom and Dad decided to help our neighbors (and best friends), Jackie and Bob Pontseele, cook all the food for their oldest daughter's high school graduation party. They worked together for days to prepare many dishes, including meatballs and mushroom gravy. After rolling out hundreds of meatballs, everyone felt a sense of accomplishment as they lined up to wash their hands. Mom discovered, to her horror, one of the rubies in her ring was missing! Where to look? Maybe it was in an aisle in the grocery store, in the parking lot…or in the meatballs. Immediately, my dad made a plan. He called a doctor friend for advice. Mush up all of the meatballs to look for it? Throw it all away just to be on the safe side? The doctor assured him that the size of the ruby in question would not cause any digestive trouble even if someone did eat it, which was highly unlikely. The graduation party went off without a hitch, and nobody found the ruby. We still laugh about how our collective parents got six daughters (between the two families) to *not* groan or gasp when someone took a spoonful of meatballs!

A natural leader, my dad was also the rock of our family. He was the one who would get phone calls at all hours for advice, the one who would walk the aging relatives down the aisle for funeral masses, the one who had an endless supply of handkerchiefs in his pocket for when anybody, particularly my sister or I, needed them. My dad could be counted on for anything. Like the time I told him at 9:30 p.m. I needed something for school the next day, or later in my life, when more traumatic events occurred (but that's another story). He might not have been happy about the situation, but he always made sure we all had what we needed. Life's little interruptions never seemed to bother my dad.

Dad taught us the importance of doing a good job. "If you don't take the time to do it right the first time, when will you find the time to do it over?" was a question that frequently escaped his lips and made our eyes roll. He expected 100 percent effort no matter what we were doing. When I was young, it was my job to vacuum the house and clean my room. Dad checked the job when I was done. One time in particular I was sent to my room to clean. My dad told me he was going to check it out afterward. Having an auditor for a father did have its drawbacks, but I was up for the challenge. I cleaned for hours. Window tracks, baseboards, closet and dresser drawer pulls…done. I called him to come and investigate the job, so proud that he would not find a speck of dust anywhere. He walked in, looked around, and strode over to the clock on my wall. He ran his finger over the top ledge, turned it over, and showed me the dust! My mouth fell open. I couldn't believe I missed it. Of course, I couldn't even reach it, and he knew that. He did ultimately tell me I did a good job. I won't even elaborate about how the vacuum lines had to be straight, with neat triangles in the carpet, extending in a fan shape from where the person vacuuming was standing. (When I moved into my own house, I vacuumed in haphazard circles for a while, just because I could!) Homework or cleaning our room, we learned that Dad didn't accept mediocrity. He didn't believe in mediocrity for himself, either. I wouldn't fully realize the true nature of his incredible work ethic until many years later.

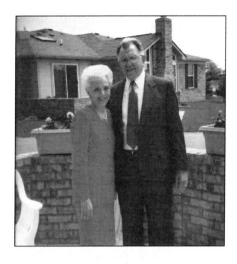

Detroit Edison hired a hardworking boy to work in the mail room. Over forty years later, he retired as a senior auditor for the company. My dad worked tirelessly to make sure that subcontractors did the work they were hired to do and that they billed the company correctly. He believed that what was right was right, and nobody was above justice. I'm sure there may have been a few happy people rejoicing on the day my dad retired, but his friends and colleagues realized what a great employee they were losing. Dad enjoyed his job very much, and I was so proud to walk next to him through the impressive foyer on the few occasions I had a reason to stop by his office.

Dad was an amazing grandpa. He would spend time taking my children for a ride across the Ambassador Bridge just to see Canada. He would take the kids to museums, air shows, and grocery shopping. He would let them help with the sausage-making but only after they washed their hands up to their armpits! One time, in jest, he told my four-year-old niece not to breathe on the meat. A few minutes later, her babushka-covered head turned toward me and her poor little face was purple! He would take them to visit family members while I was at work. He always had a comfy lap from which to listen to more stories. An army veteran, he always had stories from when he was in the service. We would later learn that his years of service would entitle him to the financial benefits that would allow him to live a full life in his home.

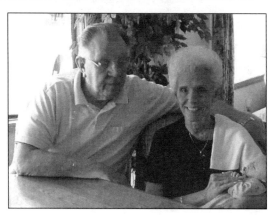

PASSING THE TORCH

Just as the Olympic Torch is passed from runner to runner, there comes a time in each family when the children grow up and slowly take over the duties that once belonged to their parents. As both of my parents got older and Dad was diagnosed with ALS, it became clear to me that the roles were changing, and I would become the caretaker. I was happy to do it, but I wasn't ready for the torch. I was still relatively young. I couldn't take over the matriarchal responsibilities of a family, even our little corner of the family. But I love to cook and entertain as well, so it was fun cooking and having my parents come to my house. Over time, as it became more difficult for Dad to walk, we began taking dinner to them. I still felt like I wasn't ready or able to take this torch. I was part of the generation raising kids and caring for aging or sick parents at the same time, so life was pretty busy.

My sister, Ann, and her family moved to Utah six months before Dad was diagnosed, so the everyday errands, necessities, and requests were my responsibility. I know that Ann was torn about going to Utah and moving so far away from the family. She and her husband had a wonderful career opportunity out there…but so far away? We all encouraged them to go and pursue their dream. I later would wonder if she blamed us for her far proximity. I, during my own moments of weakness and fear, would become very jealous of her for the same reason.

Every time it was time for my sister to go home from a visit here, I could see, through her tears, her mind wondering if this would be the last time she'd see our parents. I'm sure she was grateful for the opportunity to get "back to normal." I also know she missed our parents and worried every time the phone rang whether someone was sick, an accident had happened, or if it would entail making airline reservations to come in and help out or say final good-byes.

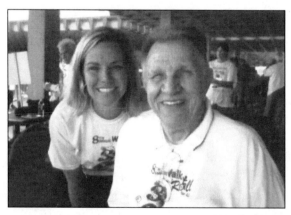

September 2010—Ann and Dad, with Mom in the background, at one of the yearly ALS of Michigan walks in which we participate.

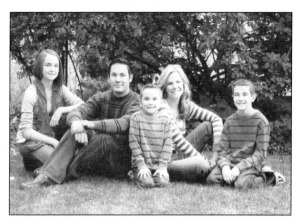

Ann's family from left to right: Lauren, Jason, Jacob, Ann, and Joseph.

ALS OF MICHIGAN AND HENRY FORD HOSPITAL— ANGELS AMONG US

I wish I had never met the ALS folks. I wish I never knew about fund-raising walks. In fact, the first time I attended an ALS walk, I cried the entire three miles. I couldn't believe how many people were there, affected by the disease, and encircling *me* with hugs and words of support and encouragement. It was overwhelming. I was invited to support group meetings where I was an absolute wreck. Seeing other people with ALS and their families going along with their daily lives, taking one day at a time sent me into panic mode. I couldn't do this. What would happen next? How could everyone be so happy when there was (and still is) no cure? How could I ever attend a meeting for newly diagnosed families and offer them any kind of support when I couldn't keep my own eyes dry? My mind wouldn't process it. If there could ever be a good thing to come out of this diagnosis, it is that with it, you become a member of the ALS family. You are welcomed into the most supportive, loving, encouraging, and caring family around.

The folks at ALS of Michigan (www.alsofmi.org) are truly angels in human form. They provided equipment from their loan closet such as a bed tray, portable ramps, power recliner, and power wheelchair, and all with the complexity of a simple phone call and a promise to return it at a later date "when you don't need it anymore." The ALS folks knew that they could give freely of their equipment. They knew that it would be returned. Once a family enters into the ALS family, they are forever changed. They usually return not only what they borrowed, but whatever else they acquired along the way. And ALS families don't usually need items for very long.

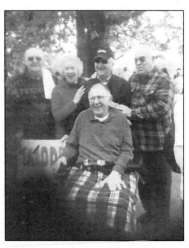

September 2011—Another ALS of Michigan walk with our wonderful family! Left to right: Al, June, Stan, Bob, and Dad.

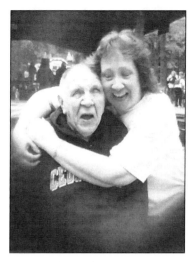

Dad and Terese "Fave"

Our family became involved in a study through Henry Ford Hospital in Detroit, Michigan. Dr. Newman, my dad's neurologist, headed a team of professionals who met with us once every three months to perform tests on Dad's lungs, muscle strength, and mobility. Ann and I attended a few meetings, but in the beginning, it was mostly Mom who attended with him. With each meeting, we could see how his numbers dropped. Less strength. Less mobility. Always lots of lung capacity though. We always said he was pretty full of hot air! After the first few meetings, the doc said Dad's ALS seemed to be "a slow mover." Some forms, the doctor explained, seemed to begin from the inside out, affecting eating, speaking, and breathing right away while my dad's form, the slow mover, seemed to work its way from the hands and feet toward the center of the body.

A slow mover. We thought that was such a blessing. At least it won't be swift and violent. Maybe there'll even be a cure in time to save him. At least we'll have him for a good long while even though the average life span after diagnosis was less than five years. We'll have time to really appreciate each other and enjoy our family.

And we did. All of our moments together became precious. There was no time for silly arguments because we had a finite amount of time together. Suddenly the unimportant stuff really was unimportant, and life's regular interruptions *were* only minor annoyances.

The folks at Henry Ford Hospital helped us get adaptive equipment to make functioning at home a little easier. They facilitated getting a mattress with an air pump to help avoid bedsores caused from being in one spot too long and not being able to move or get comfortable. Hand splints, a transfer board, compression boots for after my dad stopped walking, and a CPAP machine that helped push air into his lungs at night were items that we acquired through Ford Hospital.

PLAYING CHESS
WITH THE DEVIL

During the time from 2005 through 2012, my dad's ALS symptoms continued to worsen. Mike, our cousin, stepped in to help care for my dad. He, along with my dad's two brothers, Len and Stan, built a ramp in the garage so Dad could get in and out of the house in his wheelchair. The ramp was built by Mike and my dad's brother, Uncle Stan. Everyone else, along with a few older neighbors, stood around and supervised! I was amazed and so deeply touched that they would spend so much time to do that for my dad. It was at that time that the Sunday dinner tradition was born. Uncle Stan, and anyone else who wanted to join us, came for dinner just about every Sunday from that time forward. The conversation was always a comedy with good-hearted banter between my dad, his two brothers Len and Stan, and Mike. My mom and I would enjoy sitting and listening, laughing and shaking our heads, and eventually getting in on the fun. Our family became very close during that time. Our Sunday dinners became something everyone looked forward to. After my uncle Len passed away, the dinners continued with fond memories of what he would have said had he been there. Our Sunday dinner tradition still continues today.

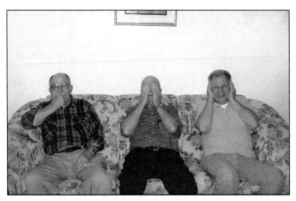

The three brothers: Len, Stan, and Jerry. Sister Elsie was, I'm sure, looking down from heaven, smiling at the brothers she affectionately called "The Three Stooges."

I later learned that Dad was Mike's hero growing up, taking him hunting, spending time at Mike's family's home, and being the "cool uncle" that many families have. Because I was going through a divorce at the time, he was like a knight in shining armor coming in to help me on the front lines. Eventually, Mike came to live with my children and me, holding down the fort while I worked full-time teaching my fourth graders and running back and forth to Dad's multiple times a day.

Mike is a master inventor. A modification here, an adjustment there. When my dad couldn't hold his cigarettes anymore, Mike fashioned a safer alternative for him. We'd light his cigarettes and tell him, "You know, those cigarettes will kill you." He'd just look up and smile an ironic smile at us. For my dad, smoking was what he enjoyed, and though the reports tell us how dangerous cigarettes can be, my dad chose to live his last years doing something he enjoyed, and we weren't going to take that away from him.

It seemed that just when Mike would figure out a way to make him more comfortable or simply able to function better, the disease would affect some other body part. When my dad couldn't remain comfortable in his bed throughout the night because his arms would fall to his side or his knees would roll toward the edges of the bed, Mike purchased a six-inch-wide piece of tubular foam, cut it in half lengthwise, and laid it on either side of him, down the full length of his body. That seemed to tuck him in well enough that he didn't have to rely on muscle strength to keep his arms in place or keep pressure off his knees. When his feet became sore from sitting in his wheelchair and being unable to shift the pressure from his ankles, Mike purchased a piece of dense foam and cut out a place for his feet to rest so they were not pressing on the footrest. When Dad's arm kept falling off the arm of the wheelchair, Mike attached a piece of plastic cutting board to the outside of the arm, creating a short "wall" to keep my dad's arm in place. When my dad lost all of the strength in his leg muscles and couldn't keep his knees from falling open, Mike came to the rescue again, this time with a soft, flat belt that would keep his knees comfortably in place without cutting into his legs. Every day, it seemed, became a modification day.

On September 23, 2008, the Department of Veteran's Affairs (DVA or VA) determined that ALS was a service-connected disability. If you or your loved one is a veteran with ALS, please check with your local ALS chapter, the Department of Veteran's Affairs, and organizations like Paralyzed Veterans of America. They will be able to help acquire financial and other benefits that will be necessary as the disease progresses.

Through the VA, my dad received funding to do some extensive remodeling on his condo. They came in and determined the modifications that would be necessary for a power wheelchair to safely move around the house. He received a ceiling lift, bathroom remodel, exit ramp, and many other modifications that made it possible for him to remain in his home.

Through all of these modifications and days that stretched into weeks, months, and years, I became angry at the disease. On my weakest days where I felt completely powerless to fix this for my dad, I would cry and tell Mike that it felt like we were playing chess with the devil. I felt like there was an evil force plotting for the next modification before we even got the current one in place. That is how the devil works though—weaving in and out of life like a silent, slithering snake, picking away at the very infrastructure of a person's faith, and creating small, incessant situations that make a person wonder if God exists at all. Why would He allow someone so wonderful to get such a horrendous disease? Why does it seem that mean and hurtful jerks live long lives in which they flourish? My dad certainly didn't ask for this through his own free will. He never did anything that would warrant such a torturous end to his life. God does work in mysterious ways though. Maybe he had lessons to learn. Maybe we all did.

It is interesting. Knowing the theoretical steps of the grieving process doesn't really mean anything until you live it. Reading about the fact that this process applies not only to death, but any form of loss made sense, but didn't really sink in. Knowing I would be facing the steps of denial, anger, depression, and acceptance didn't really mean anything until I was standing in the middle of the grocery store and memories of shopping with my dad flooded over me, sending the waterworks into high gear. Or going alone to an Easter basket food blessing service, a ritual that was exclusively my dad's and mine. I cried in the parking lot for so long that I missed it. I couldn't do all of those things alone. My dad was always one of my greatest supporters. He was calm and patient, and he always had the best advice—whether we wanted to hear it or not! My dad was such a strong, proud man, and there he was, stuck back at the house in his power wheelchair. Worse yet, his mind was as sharp as ever, and he *knew* all of the things he couldn't do anymore. He saw every day the decline in his ability to even care for himself. I truly learned that the grieving process didn't occur only after a person dies. Again, I knew that any traumatic situation could set it in motion, but I didn't *really learn* it until then.

Unfortunately, Dad discovered what he could and couldn't do through accidents like falling, getting stuck on the stairs, or getting stuck midway through transferring himself to the bed or the toilet because he was too tired to continue or his muscles just plain wouldn't work. Dad knew that his trips to the family Fourth of July party were over when he tripped on a short stair and broke his ankle. We stood around, helpless to move him and get him comfortable. Finally, some muscular cousins heaved him up and onto a chair. Another particularly traumatic day occurred while Dad was cooking hard-boiled eggs so Mom could rest. He was moving the tiny pot with two eggs over to the sink, and his arm gave out midway. The pot of boiling water tipped, and the boiling water landed in his lap. It took two trips to the hospital, about two pounds of silver sulfadiazine cream applied like cake frosting, and months to heal, as his body was so busy fighting the ALS. Of course, the scars were permanent.

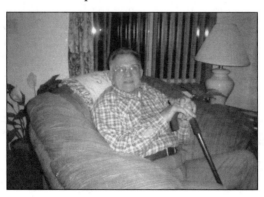

2004—Still smiling!

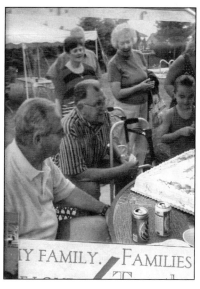

July 2005—Happy Seventieth birthday, Dad! So many
friends and family members came to celebrate with us!

Stress—After a While, Even Holding Empty Arms Up Is Difficult

There was a story I read once about a woman who walked into a lecture hall holding a half-full glass of water, ready to give a talk about stress. The audience assumed she would begin with the customary half-full/half-empty question, when she asked, "How heavy is this glass of water?" The audience, surprised, threw out some numbers. She explained that even a small glass of water becomes unbearably heavy when held up over one's head for an extended period of time. She discussed the importance of being able to set your stress down, step away from it, and return refreshed and ready to deal with it again another time.

Similarly, during one of my undergraduate classes, we participated in an activity simulating a family with a special needs child. The special needs person was in the center of a group of four, who represented the family of caregivers surrounding him or her. While the person in the middle stood still, the caregivers were all asked to raise their right arm and touch fingers with the other caregivers over the special needs person's head. We were then asked to slowly walk in a circle around the special needs person. We were asked to pay attention to the point at which we began to feel tired or in pain. It was amazing how difficult that simulation was. Almost immediately, we became tired. Our arms eventually lost circulation. We began tripping over our own feet.

Sometimes, during the longest days, my prayers would be simply to make it through the day to bedtime. It wasn't even the physical stress of running back and forth taking meals, feeding, or putting my dad to bed. Sometimes it was the worrying that caused the most stress. Worrying about my parents being alone for the whole night. Worrying about my mother and whether or not she would be able to handle the things that my dad may need during the night...or during the day...or...or...

As stressed out as I was, I was so grateful for Mike, our extended family members, and other folks who came in to care for Dad. ALS of Michigan provided a few hours of respite care every week. During that time, a nurse would come in and bathe him, change his bedding, and perform other personal care tasks. I was so grateful to be able to put the stress down for short amounts of time.

When Mom's health declined and she could no longer go with Dad to his doctor appointments, Mike stepped in again. He took Dad downtown for his appointments and then took him for a ride or to the casino. Dad couldn't reach out to play the slot machines but still enjoyed the atmosphere. Even after he was diagnosed, Dad took Mom to the casino about once a month. They would go with their very good friends, Rose Marie and Chuck. Friends from high school, Rose Marie and Mom were always extremely close and shared many conversations throughout the years about their husbands, growing families, and how to fix the world's problems. After Chuck passed away, Rose Marie continued to keep in close contact and visited Mom and Dad whenever she could, especially if they could work their plans around a short casino trip!

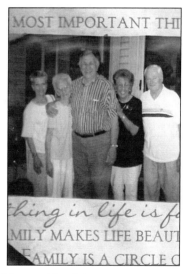

Some of Mom and Dad's best friends from high school, left to right: Rose Marie, Mom, Dad, Karen, and Kevin. Rose Marie's husband, Chuck, was enjoying the party from heaven.

Mom was a great caregiver. She helped my dad all she could, which was sometimes not a whole lot due to her heart condition and her own ailing health. They took their caregiving responsibilities for each other very seriously. I never realized how scary the situation must have been for her. She had always been the one that was *taken care of*. She was the one with the long-term heart condition. After my dad's diagnosis trumped her illness, I'm sure it was hard for her to switch both mentally and physically to that of the role of caregiver. I'm sure it took a serious toll on her health.

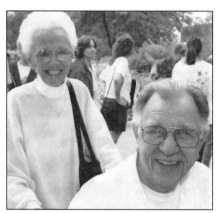

Another ALS of Michigan walk and *still smiling*!

One afternoon I received a phone call from Dad. "Can you come over? Your mother's not breathing well. She doesn't want to go, but I think she should go to the hospital." Of course, I sped over at once. Living just a mile apart did have its perks! When I got to the house, Mom was sitting up and breathing very quickly and shallowly. "Mom, I'm calling 911 so they can bring the oxygen and professionals to you instead of trying to drive you to the hospital myself." She didn't argue. That was the first sign that her situation was dire. Mom hated going to the hospital. She couldn't smoke there. More importantly, she couldn't be around to make sure Dad was okay.

One never gets over the adrenaline rush of having to talk to 911 operators. Though I sounded calm, I was a nervous wreck inside! When the paramedics got to the house, they immediately hooked Mom up to oxygen and got her on the stretcher. I became panicked when they waited for my dad to align his wheelchair next to her so he could give her a kiss. I kept thinking they were wasting precious time…go! Get her to the hospital! They must have known. They gave Dad time to give her a final kiss good-bye though he didn't know it then.

Mom was admitted to the hospital. The next morning, I received a call from hospice. They wanted to admit her. Hospice!?! The word sent chills up my spine. Ann flew into town, and we signed the papers, crying the whole time. We brought Dad up to the hospital to say good-bye, and she received the sacrament of Anointing of the Sick with our family around her. Ann and I stayed with her through the night, each one of us holding one of her hands and leaning our heads on her bed while we all slept. Ann is a nurse who spent part of her career working at an oncology office. She was used to working with terminal patients, but it's different when it's your own mother. At 3:36 a.m., Ann and I fully awoke when Mom squeezed our hands with a strength we had *never* known her to have. I looked up to her chest in anticipation of her next labored breath…and there simply was none. In what seemed like slow motion, I reached up gently to feel her neck for a pulse or movement of air, and I couldn't feel anything. Ann started yelling, "MOM!"

I said quietly, "She's gone." I believe she woke us to let us know she was leaving and to let us know she loved us. I called Mike, who was spending the night with Dad. I think Dad knew as soon as the phone rang.

The next days passed in a blur. Funeral arrangements, contacting family and friends, and trying to help Dad rest were our top priorities. He was such a trooper. No longer able to move his arms, let alone walk, he needed help wiping his nose at the funeral. In an ironic turn of events, I stood by him, wiping his tears with his own handkerchief as they freely fell.

I know losing Mom shattered Dad's heart. I know he missed her from the very bottom of his heart. I think he was relieved that she was out of pain, that she didn't have to care for him anymore, and that he didn't have to worry about her anymore either. He always had such a sense of responsibility when it came to Mom. I think he also worried about his own future too. He wasn't sure what would happen next or who would take care of *him*. He seemed to decline much faster after Mom died. Whether it was the disease, his sense that *his* caretaking job was finished, or his general will to live, I can't say.

I immediately went into "Dad mode." I put my grief aside and concentrated fully on things that Dad needed. I liked it that way. I preferred it, in fact. I didn't have to deal with losing my mother, and I put all my effort into trying to fill my dad's shoes and be his rock.

As Dad's body continued to fight this exhausting disease, my children stepped in to help. My oldest son, David, moved in with Grandpa and helped him out for over a year. He helped with daily tasks, nighttime needs, and basically put his whole twenty-year-old life on hold to care for the grandfather who helped raise him when he was a baby. Life really does come full circle.

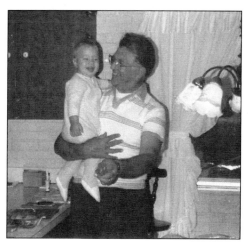

The bond between David and Grandpa was immediate.
They were among each other's very favorite people.

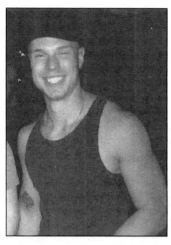

Dave grew into a strong, caring young man who then took care of Grandpa. They were still among each other's very favorite people.

David and I became closer during the time he cared for his grandpa. We would have late-night chats on my patio after Dave put Grandpa to bed. Mostly he wanted to know what would happen next. The stress of being a twenty-year-old caregiver was getting to him, and he didn't know how to alleviate it. He didn't want to desert Grandpa, but he felt like he was in the thick, never-ending fog too. "Mom, how long is this going to go on? What's going to happen next?" I told him that all we can do is take things one day at a time and do the best we can do. So much for Mom having all the answers! Shortly thereafter, I'm sure as part of God's plan, we found out about another caregiver who was looking for a place to live. We knew him, and my dad was comfortable with him.

He moved in with Dad, and David moved out into his own house. I was so proud of how David stayed with Grandpa until the natural progression of the disease required a more skilled caregiver. That part of God's plan seemed to work out perfectly.

As Dad's disease continued to worsen and he continued to need more skilled care, it became necessary to make yet another plan. We were forever "making another plan." We began a series of coverage shifts that included all four of my children giving up time that they could have otherwise spent to sit with Grandpa. The kids, David (twenty), Jeff (sixteen), Andy (fourteen), and Katie (ten) knew about Grandpa's disease and that his time with us was limited. They looked forward to "Grandpa sitting." We talked about the fact that this time with him is precious and would be something they could look back on after he was gone. Nobody ever complained about going to Grandpa's. I was so proud of them because they took their jobs seriously and learned about what a special man their grandpa was. They would also learn that, in their mourning, they would be comforted knowing that they were instrumental in making his last months of life more comfortable and happy. They learned at a young age the value of unconditional love; that sometimes we can't offer a solution to a problem, but we can make the days more tolerable for someone. Sometimes just being there with a person is what makes it most tolerable. It is one of life's most important lessons.

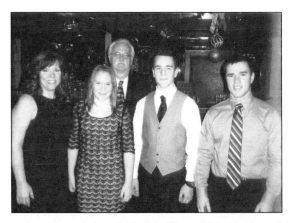

December 2012—left to right: Me, Katie, Mike, Andy, and Jeff

We learned so much about unconditional love. When it became clear that our system of tucking Dad into bed at night, arranging his phone, emergency button, TV remote, and urinal didn't work anymore because he couldn't be alone for more than a few hours, we asked Dad again to come and live with us. He was concerned that he would become "a burden" to us and that the kids didn't need a sick Grandpa around. On the contrary, dear Dad. That was absolutely what they needed. They needed to see that this is how we care for and rally around our family members. We help them and do whatever we can to make them more comfortable. Not only that, but I wanted my dad to live with us because it would ease *my* worrying about being away from him. I could look over while cooking dinner and make sure he was okay. I could hear him yell if he needed me during the night. I could squeeze every last drop of conversation and family history out of him! I was comforted in the fact that he would be right there and checking on him wouldn't require a car ride to his condo. During our conversation, I also mentioned that one day *I* would be old and in need of care, and I wanted my children to know what to do! It was only after believing that he was helping teach lessons to us that he consented to come and live with us. Construction in my front room started immediately.

As much as I loved spending time with my dad and being the one to kiss his forehead after tucking him in for the night, there were times I longed to trade places with my sister, who had a "normal" life back in Utah. Ann and her family came in two or three times a year, as much as they could. Along with missing her, I found myself jealous of the fact that they could pick up and leave this situation and return to their daily life. I knew in my heart that I truly didn't want to trade places with her and that she probably just as desperately wanted to stay, but terminal diseases can do crazy things to a person's thinking.

ATTITUDE

Philosophers say that life is 3 percent about what happens to us and 97 percent about how we deal with and adjust to it. Dad had the attitude of the richest man in the world. Amazingly, he smiled whenever anyone was around. I don't know what went on in his mind when he was alone, but I never, in all nine years of dealing with this disease, saw him angry, disappointed, or depressed. He was happy to welcome anyone into his home, and even when he couldn't get his guests food or drinks, he would send them to the fridge, calling out the names of available food and drink choices.

Dad had an "attitude of gratitude" and a thank-you for everyone with whom he crossed paths. Whether it was someone coming in to help him, or the lady at the grocery store, there was always time for a little chat. He consistently thanked everyone who took the time to come and see or call him before they left or hung up. He truly appreciated all the good in his life, from his wife and two daughters, to his extended family, friends, clergy, and health-care professionals. He respected most everyone and was deeply respected in return.

Going downtown to Henry Ford Hospital every three months turned into a small party. We would walk in to heartfelt greetings, be escorted to a room, and spend about the next three hours meeting with everyone from the speech pathologist, to the occupational therapist, physical therapist, neurologist, a representative from the national ALS Association (www.alsa.org), respiratory therapist, nutritionist, psychologist, and faith services representatives. Everyone loved when Dad would come in. They all remarked about how incredible he was and how much fun their job could be (given the terminal nature of their patients). They genuinely loved him, and he felt the same way about them. If he needed a piece of equipment, they made sure it was ordered and on its way immediately. The staff called to check up on him even during the in-between times. To show his appreciation, he sent flowers to the office every Christmas, and many times took candy in when he had a scheduled appointment.

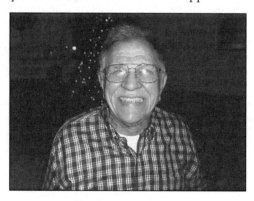

Here's a smile for you!

LOSING THE BATTLE

"Courage isn't always a lion's roar. It is sometimes the heart at the end of the day saying, 'I will try again tomorrow.'" (Mary Anne Radmacher). From the time Mom died in 2010, either the disease seemed to move more quickly, or Dad was just getting tired of fighting it. His attitude was still great, especially given the circumstances, but we could see it in his eyes that he was getting tired. On Wednesday, June 15, 2012, Dad went into the hospital for the last time. He hadn't been able to "get under" and clear his cough for about a month. His lungs were filling up, and he no longer had the strength to cough and clear his airway.

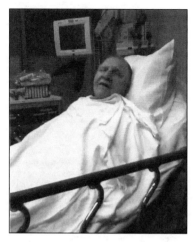

June 15, 2012—The day before Dad died, and he was *still smiling*!

Dad's oxygen levels were off, and he was hallucinating, seeing objects floating in the air. He seemed to be lost in a delusional world, not knowing what was real and what was his imagination. At one point, Dad looked at the ceiling with fear in his eyes, and asked me, "Are those things on the ceiling real?" When I assured him there was nothing there, he looked confused at first, then relieved. He never mentioned what he thought he saw. After Mike and I left that night, the nurse called me. She said Dad was being combative, refusing a bath. I asked her to let it go for the night. It had become so painful for my dad when we moved him around, that the thought of people rolling him to his side for a bath probably scared him, and he was not going to have any part of that! It wasn't worth his agitation.

WORLDS APART

Meanwhile, across the country, my sister Ann and her family were on the way to the Las Vegas airport preparing to take a family vacation of a lifetime to Europe. After speaking to the doctors, she informed her husband, Jason, and their kids that they would be flying that day, but not to Europe. The plan had changed, and they would be flying to Michigan to say good-bye to Grandpa.

My sister arrived on a Thursday night after catching the last plane of the day to Detroit Metropolitan Airport. She raced through the airport, crying, and begging the people in the long line at security to please let her through. "My father is dying in Michigan, and I have to get on this plane." They sent her through to the front of the line without question. Jason and the kids arrived on Friday afternoon. At that point, we were discussing hospice options. Dad, the patriarch, was asking *my* advice. "Julie, what should I do? I guess this is the end, eh?"

"Dad, we can sign you into inpatient hospice and help control your pain. Then, if we decide to, we can sign you out again."

"Okay, let's do it." I think he knew he wouldn't be coming out of hospice, but he wanted to spare me the burden of making the hospice decision. I think I also knew he wouldn't be coming out of hospice, but I couldn't admit it. I would absolutely fall apart.

SLIPPING AWAY

Waiting for the hospice papers to clear was pure torture. Thankfully, we had the support of our childhood friends, the Pontseeles, to give us strength. My friend Julie and her sister Denise, our best friends from the time we could walk and part of the meatball/ruby escapade, were there with us to sign him into hospice, and they didn't leave our side for the entire day. We cried together along with each doctor that came in to examine Dad. They knew the look of a patient as the body begins to shut down. They know the sound of the "death rattle" when the lung function becomes inefficient, and all they could do was be there with us. There were no comforting words, but it was so comforting that they were there, sharing their own humanness and vulnerability with us.

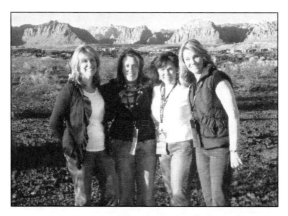

2009—The Girls' Utah Trip. From left to right: Julie, Denise, Me, and Ann. Though Julie and Denise are now happily married, they will always be "The Pontseele Girls." The other Pontseele sisters, Kim and Renee, couldn't make the trip this time.

It was at that time that I made the phone call to the number on the card that I'd carried in my wallet for years. "Please Call When Death Is Imminent." My dad made the decision, when he was first diagnosed, to donate his brain and spinal column to the ALS Bio Repository Clinic upon his death. He believed deeply that researchers were close to unlocking the mysteries of the disease, and he wanted to be part of the research. Even after death, my dad was a tremendously selfless person. Talk about a guy giving you the shirt off his back… or his brain. He was a strong believer in organ donation too. I remember sitting in my dad's hospice room talking with my brother-in-law about the bio Repository program and, after reading the card to him, asking, "When is death imminent?"

"Now."

I made the call and got the arrangements in motion.

There comes a time when your prayers change. In that moment, they changed from, "Please help the doctors find a cure for this disease in enough time that it will save my dad" to "Please, Lord, take him quickly and gently. Please end his suffering and bring him home to Mom and your eternal love." As much as I would miss him, I prayed this prayer with all my heart.

I believe doctors always want to do what's best for their patients. The doctors and nurses were amazing. When Dad was on the "hospital" track, the focus was on getting better and going home. As a result, medications were carefully monitored and regulated. When he was moved to the "hospice" track, the focus shifted to pain management and comfort. The doctors and nurses continued to support our family during this transition time, even though there was nothing physically they could do to bring Dad's health back. Again, just being there together, throughout the natural process of death, was an important life lesson for all of us. Hospice nurses are some of the strongest people I have come to know.

The twelve or so hours between the time we signed Dad into hospice and the time he was officially admitted to hospice were agonizing. It was heart-wrenching to watch Dad struggle to breathe, watching him slowly drown in the lung secretions associated with this final stage of ALS, and knowing that one of his two most secret and most traumatizing fears, the fear of fire and the fear of drowning, was materializing right before my eyes, and I was helpless to rescue him.

Good-Bye

Once again, Ann and I spent the night at the hospital. The hospice staff kept Dad comfortable with their pain management concoctions. When Dad would become restless or begin to appear uncomfortable, the nurses were there immediately with relief-giving medicine. It was a long night, sitting next to Dad, waiting for his next breath.

Morning broke, June 17, 2012, and he was still hanging on. We had short amounts of time when he was awake, but he slept for the most part. When Ann went down to get us some coffee, I held Dad's hand and began talking to him. "Happy Father's Day, Dad. I'm so proud of you and how you have fought this fight. You're tired now. Please don't worry about Ann and me. We'll be fine. It is time for you to go home to heaven and see Mom. You just go whenever you're ready." I think he was waiting for me to say that.

Family and friends gathered from near and far. Dad's great-niece, Melissa, who had become one of his caregivers, came in along with her daughter Alex. They wanted to wish Dad a happy Father's Day and give him a hug. Meanwhile, across town, Teresa, the niece he called "Fave," was on her way to the airport to pick up her daughter, who had recently graduated from Coast Guard Basic Training after she received a special release to come to Michigan and say good-bye. They wouldn't make it in time.

My dad's friend Jack Heitchue came to say good morning. Jack had been to visit Dad every Friday morning for years to pray with him and give him Holy Communion. Dad looked forward to Jack's visits, requesting plates of cookies or snacks be put out for him. I am so grateful to Jack for the time he spent with Dad, praying with him and talking with him about his spirituality and all of those other things longtime friends (not "old" friends!) talk about. Jack told Dad good-bye, and we cried together. We knew it would not be much longer.

Bob and Jackie Pontseele, our "second set of parents," came in next. They prayed with us, cried, reminisced, and sat with Dad. Just when Bob began telling us how proud he was of us, Dad opened his shining green eyes and looked at us. For a long moment, time stood still. His look reminded me of the very first look a newborn baby gives its mother. All-encompassing and full of wonder. Ann and I were once again on either side of him, hugging him, and crying. As he took his last breath, peacefulness set over the room on that Father's Day afternoon, and I believe it was the perfect day for him to go home to our Heavenly Father.

ORPHANS

The emotional highs and lows following the days of a loved one's death cause our memories to blur. It is an odd, empty feeling when you realize that both of your parents are gone, and it's all up to you. I officially had the torch. I have been given the responsibility of carrying on family traditions for the younger generation; I am responsible to give the advice that they may ask for, and the people to whom I have turned for my whole life are not there anymore.

The funeral home was the same one where Mom was laid out. The folks at Lee Elena Funeral Home in Macomb, Michigan, were so gracious throughout those days. We couldn't have asked for more support or comfort during the times we needed someone to have clear heads in order to make the arrangements. Another cousin, Tom, Uncle Stan's son, who worked at the funeral home, worked on both Mom and Dad. It was comforting knowing that even during their final preparations they were surrounded by family.

Because Dad was an army veteran, he was entitled to a full military send-off. Representatives from the VFW came out to perform the service, including a moving twenty-one-gun salute. My cousin, Kayla, who had just graduated from Coast Guard Basic Training, and had missed seeing him at the hospital before he died, surprised everyone by participating in the service. After finding out about the death in the family, her supervisors shipped her formal uniform to Michigan so she could participate in the service. As you can imagine, there wasn't a dry eye in the room. We were so proud of her courage, and I have the flag that she personally folded and handed to me during the service. It is proudly on display in my great room where we can see it all day long.

After the service, I stood up to thank those who attended, and I was shocked at the huge number of people I saw. People filled the room and spilled out into the main hallways. "Thank you so much for coming and being part of my dad's beautiful service. We appreciate your support over the last years, and we invite you to join us in the hospitality room for some drinks and snacks. You know how my dad was, and you know that he would not let you leave without eating and drinking something!" A chorus of laughs erupted as we all traveled to the hospitality room together, laughing at various fond memories of him, and talking about how beautiful and moving the ceremony was.

As I looked around and saw our closest friends and family enjoying snacks and drinks, I was struck by the absolute joyous atmosphere in the room. Again, time stood still, as I imagined what the scene must look like to an onlooker standing above.

Dad! I had forgotten about him for a minute. Panicked, I walked down the hall to the room where he was. It was completely empty. At first I felt badly for him; we all left him to go eat. But then, as I approached the casket, a feeling of pride set in. I leaned down and whispered, "Dad, there is a beautiful party going on in there. It is just how you would have wanted it. Everyone is laughing, eating, and drinking. I know you're looking down on us and smiling. Thank you for your gift of loving to entertain."

Life is about human interaction. It is in the interruptions of life that God's agenda interrupts our own. It may be there in those interruptions that we come to know more fully of God's grace and love. They are challenges that can profoundly change our lives. They are invitations to learn, grow, change, and heal.

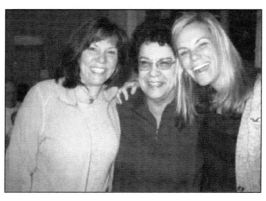

Our "second Mom," Jackie Pontseele, with Ann and me. Mr. Pontseele, our "second Dad," was in the background rocking his granddaughter.

CHECKMATE

The mass was beautiful, just like I knew it would be. The luncheon was a carbon copy of Mom's, at Dad's request, and we were sitting down, preparing to eat. Ann spoke about coming in to see Dad and some of the things she felt and experienced during his illness.

It was my turn to address the roomful of people who had come together because my dad had touched their lives in some way or another. I had no idea what to say to them. I began, "My story is a bit different from Ann's. Throughout the years, particularly the last few, I have told Mike so many times that this disease was like playing chess with the devil. It seemed that every time we successfully modified something, the disease would progress and require another modification. I think demonizing the disease gave me something at which to be mad. It wasn't until today, surrounded by all of you, that I realize that Dad triumphed over the disease and all of the evil things it did to his body. He is in heaven with Mom and the Lord. His pain is gone, and he knows God's ultimate grace and love. He got his wings. He won the game."

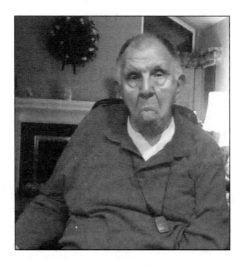

Checkmate.

Afterward

I am grateful to the Lord for bringing my dad home to heaven. I am grateful that he is with Mom, and they are again watching over each other and living with God. They fulfilled the goals that the rest of us hope to reach one day. I don't know what heaven looks like, but I can only imagine that it is a beautiful place, filled with love, peace, service to others, and gratitude. Fear, sickness, and sadness are nonexistent. I am so happy I don't have to worry about them and their earthly bodies. I am comforted in the knowledge that they continue to be exactly where God wants them.

That being said, I'm so lonely without them that some days it's hard to keep my brain occupied. So many times I've wanted to share some great news about the kids, share something that happened that only they could fully appreciate, or ask for the advice that I haven't always enthusiastically received in the past. Even now, months later, I think of my dad every time I go to the store because that was our routine for so long. Every time one of the kids wins an award, gets a good grade on something they worked hard for, or reaches a new milestone, I want to call him. Sometimes I will think of some juicy piece of gossip that my dad would appreciate and then realize that he's not there to answer the phone. It is like being in the twilight zone sometimes. I have learned that the reason that God gave me two parents is because I couldn't do this a third time. Caring for, burying, and grieving the loss of your parents takes a lot out of you! We attend funerals for grandparents, other extended family members, spouses, and devastatingly, children; but nowhere in there is the circle of life as poignant as when you bury the very people who gave you life.

The time has come for us to create a new "normal." Everyday tasks remain the same, but different. The kids will continue to do well in their work and school goals. They'll continue to have band and choir concerts. We'll continue to be a karate family, training and testing for our next belt rank and attending the many functions the dojo hosts. I'll continue to teach and write, but it won't be the same without my parents. We'll continue to have Sunday dinner with Uncle Stan, who has become more and more like a father figure for me, and anyone else who wants to join us. (Give me a call…we'll set an extra plate!) We'll continue to celebrate holidays at our house, carrying on the traditions that my parents started, and some they passed down from *their* parents.

This past December 2012, we celebrated our first Christmas without Mom and Dad. I truly didn't know how I was going to fare. I was dreading our traditional Christmas Eve celebration as much as I would have dreaded walking over hot coals. Was I going to burst into tears when the first guest showed up? Was I going to even be able to get out of bed that day? I could only busy myself with food and gift preparations and trust that God had it covered. Of course, he did. I purchased matching candleholders for my sister, all of the Pontseeles, Cousin Terese "Fave," and me. I sent them a note telling them of our matching candles, and asking them to please light them during their holiday celebrations, wherever and whenever they have them, as a reminder that my parents are with us no matter where we are or what we are doing. During our first Christmas Eve without them, it gave me more comfort than I expected, looking over at the two glowing tea light candles in the beautiful peace lily candleholder next to Mom and Dad's picture. Surrounded by family and special friends, the evening was full of laughter and peace. I would highly recommend lighting a special candle for any family experiencing the loss of a loved one. As sure as we saw the flickering light, we felt my parents' presence all evening. I think they would have been proud.

I attended a women's silent retreat in November 2012 along with some of the Pontseele girls and Mrs. P. We had a wonderful time and heard some very inspiring talks, particularly by Sister Janet Schaeffler, OP. She conducted a seminar about Life's Interruptions. It was her perspective that helped me to gain clarity about my dad's ALS and the life lessons that God had in store for all of us. She said that it is in those interruptions that God taps us on the shoulder and intervenes with His own master plan. We tend to be so wrapped up in our work being interrupted that we fail to realize that God's interruptions *are* our work. It is in those interruptions that God speaks to us about the things in life that are most important: faith, hope, love.

TAKEAWAYS

If you, a friend, or loved one has been diagnosed with ALS, please contact the ALS Association (www.ALSA. org). There you will find so much information regarding ALS symptoms, research updates, and local chapters. If you live in Michigan, you can also contact ALS of Michigan (www. alsofmi.org) for information, loan closet items, local support groups, and you may be able to be placed on a list to have some respite care provided at no cost to you.

The most important takeaway from this book is for you to know that you are not alone in your fight. As I said at the beginning of the book, you are part of the most supportive group of people around. Contact the ALS chapters in your area.

Accept help. If friends or loved ones offer to run errands, clean the house, do wash, or just come and sit with you or your loved one, take the help! Many hands make light work. This disease progression will become difficult enough all on its own without you trying to do everything all of the time, especially if you or your loved one has been diagnosed with the "slow mover" version, which can last years.

Plan for the future. This disease is one in which you will need to be thinking about and planning for what comes next. As much as you may not want to think about this, it is necessary because unless the secrets of this disease are unlocked soon, it will progress. Make your plans while you are still strong.

Get your financial affairs in order and designate a patient advocate. This is someone who can sign for you and/or speak for you when the time comes that you may not be able to do this for yourself. Contact a local attorney and discuss estate planning.

Make sure your wishes for your final resting place are known by your family or friends. Do you want to plan your funeral? Cremation or burial? These are difficult questions, but we'll all get there someday, even the currently healthy ones! You can pay for some of these services in advance, thereby helping out those responsible for making final arrangements. Make sure your family/planner knows what you want. It will make their planning easier, and they'll be comforted knowing that it was "as he/she wanted it."

If the ALS patient is a veteran, please contact the US Department of Veterans Affairs (www.va.gov). Veterans, depending on their length and level of service, may be entitled to financial compensation and other benefits that will become vital as the disease progresses.

Get your spiritual issues in order. Contact your local clergy members. Even if you don't practice a specific religion, you can still enrich your relationship with God. Don't believe in God? I won't tell you what to believe, but it sure made our journey more tolerable, knowing in our hearts that He put us right where we were meant to be at every given moment. You can go it alone, but know that God is waiting for you to ask His help if you choose to let Him guide your heart.

Get your relationships in order. Make those phone calls, say "I'm sorry" if you need to, say "thank you" to at least one person every day, and understand that with this diagnosis, you have been given a very special gift. You cannot take time for granted any longer. Pay attention to the beauty of the world around you. You have been given a finite amount of time in which to make any amends necessary for a peaceful transition from your earthly body. Use it well. It doesn't matter what the argument was about or whose fault it was. The better person is the one who extends the olive branch of peace. If that branch has been extended to you and you have refused it in the past, go and grab it now! You will be amazed at how much better you feel, and you will feel completely ready and at peace when the time comes.

As I have already said, the most important takeaway from this book is to know you are not alone in your fight. It is not our expertise that blesses people; it is our humanness. I thank you for sharing our journey with me, and I wish you a gentle journey.